SLIM DOWN RECIPES DIET COOKBOOK

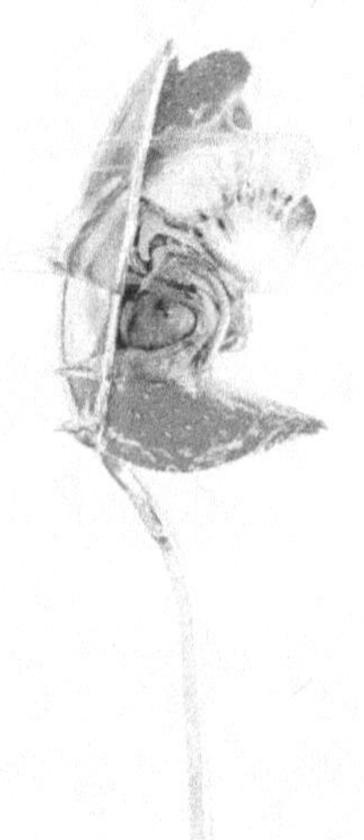

It is certain you must reduce 10 pounds in one week with my magic slimming down delicious recipes without sacrificing taste. +4 week weight management meal plan

Dr.Raymond Harris

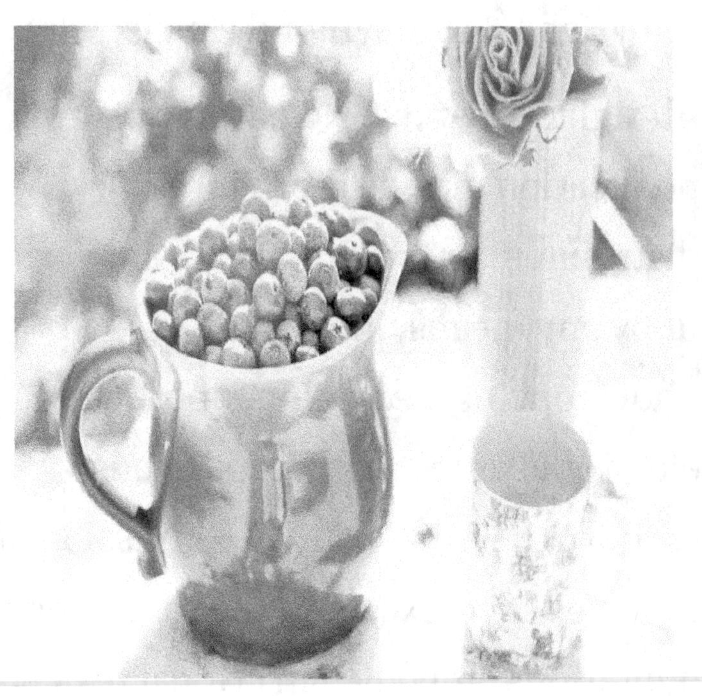

Table of content

Recipes ingredient and instruction

Chapter five
slim-down supper dishes
together with their components
and instructions:

healthful and slim-down snack
recipes together with their
components and instructions:

excellent seafood and fish dishes
together
with their components and
instructions:

Delicious meat dishes together with their ingredients and instructions:

colorful salad dishes with a range of tastes and textures

Chapter seven
wonderful dessert recipes to fulfill your sweet tooth:

Chapter one

Introduction to Slim Down Recipes

 Welcome to the world of Slim Down Recipes, as we begin on a delectable path towards a better, more vibrant living. In this chapter, we'll establish the framework for your culinary expedition.

Welcome and Overview

Discover the interesting selection of recipes that will assist you towards attaining your health and fitness objectives. Whether you're aiming to reduce a few pounds or just establish a healthier eating habit, this cookbook is your partner on this gratifying route.

Importance of a Balanced Diet
Uncover the value of having a balanced diet for general well-being. Explore how the appropriate balance of nutrients, vitamins, and minerals may significantly improve your energy levels, metabolism, and long-term health.

Understanding Portion Control
Delve into the art of portion management and understand how it

plays a critical part in controlling
weight and fostering a healthy lifestyle.
Discover practical techniques and
tactics to help you enjoy your meals
while retaining control over your
calorie consumption.

Embark on this gastronomic trip with
the knowledge and determination to
make positive changes in your diet,
setting the scene for a healthier,
happier self.

Essential Ingredients

we discuss the fundamental

components that constitute the backbone of Slim Down Recipes. From nutrient-rich ingredients to creative culinary switches and key kitchen basics, explore how these factors contribute to producing tasty and health-conscious meals.

Nutrient-Rich Foods
Dive into the world of nutrient-dense foods that carry a potent punch of vitamins, minerals, and antioxidants. Learn about the bright variety of fruits, vegetables, lean meats, and whole grains that will not only improve the taste of your food but also supply necessary nutrients to promote your well-being.

Smart Swaps for Healthier Cooking
Explore creative and health-conscious alternatives to standard ingredients and culinary techniques. From swapping refined sugars to introducing heart-healthy fats, explore a range of smart changes that enhance the nutritional content of your meals without sacrificing on flavor.

Kitchen Staples for Slimming Meals
Stock your kitchen with key items that form the basis of slimming and tasty dishes. From herbs and spices that give depth to tastes to pantry mainstays like whole grains and legumes,

learn the crucial components that
make creating healthful meals a breeze.

Equip yourself with the knowledge and
supplies required to convert your
kitchen into a hive of healthy culinary
delights. These key items will set the
setting for a delightful and satisfying
culinary experience on your quest to a
leaner, healthier lifestyle

Chapter two

Breakfast Boosters

Start your day on a healthful note with these invigorating and enjoyable breakfast alternatives. From vivid smoothie bowls to protein-packed burritos and flexible overnight oats, this chapter is a celebration of good morning sustenance.

Energizing Smoothie Bowls
Indulge in a rush of flavors and nutrition with this selection of revitalizing smoothie bowl recipes. Packed with fruits, veggies, and superfoods,

these bowls give a refreshing and healthful start to your day. Discover innovative toppings that add crunch and texture, making each bowl a pleasurable experience.

Protein-Packed Breakfast Burritos Experience the ideal balance of taste and protein with our morning burrito creations. Filled with healthy meats, colorful greens, and a range of spices, these burritos are a tasty way to jumpstart your morning. Explore numerous combinations and pick your favorite fillings for a tasty and healthful breakfast.

Overnight Oats Variations
Streamline your mornings with the ease of overnight oats. Uncover a wealth of options, from traditional combos to unique tastes that adapt to your taste preferences. Discover how basic ingredients may convert into a substantial and healthy breakfast alternative, ready to enjoy as soon as you wake up.

Revitalize your mornings with these breakfast boosters, setting the tone for a day full with energy and nutrients. These dishes indicate that a nutritious breakfast can be both tasty and quick to make, ensuring you're ready to face whatever comes your way.

Light Lunches

In this chapter, we explore various alternatives for light and fulfilling meals that will keep you energetic throughout the day. From vivid salads to veggie-packed wraps and soothing soups and stews, these dishes provide a great blend of taste and nutrition.

Colorful Salad Creations
Embrace the rainbow with this array of bright salad concoctions. Discover imaginative combinations of fresh veggies, lean meats, and healthful grains that transform a basic salad into a fulfilling and visually beautiful dinner.

From zesty sauces to creative toppings, these salads revolutionize the art of light and tasty meals.

Veggie-Packed Wraps and Sandwiches Elevate your lunchtime meal with our range of veggie-packed wraps and sandwiches. Explore imaginative combinations of bright veggies, lean meats, and savory spreads, all wrapped in your choice of whole-grain wraps or snuggled between pieces of healthy bread. These dishes alter the conventional sandwich, making it a healthful and enjoyable choice for lunch.

Satisfying Soup and Stew Recipes
Warm up your lunchtime with these soothing soup and stew dishes. Packed with nutrient-rich veggies, lean meats, and fragrant herbs, these recipes provide a satisfying and delicious alternative for a light lunch. Whether you like a comforting cup of soup or a substantial stew, these dishes are meant to feed and please.

Transform your lunch routine with these light and tasty choices. From vivid salads to satisfying wraps and warm soups, these dishes illustrate that a light lunch can be both tasty and full, supporting your health journey one bite at a time.

Wholesome Dinners

Step into the heart of healthful meals
with our selection of dishes meant to
feed and please. From lean protein
meals to fragrant vegetable stir-fries
and oven-baked delights, this chapter
provides a range of alternatives to make
your evenings both healthful and
delightful.

Lean Protein Entrées
Explore a choice of lean protein sources
that take center stage in these healthful
meals. From grilled chicken and fish to
plant-based protein sources,

these dishes offer a tasty basis for a healthy supper. Discover unique marinades and spice combinations that boost the tastes of your protein selections.

Flavorful Veggie Stir-Fries
Immerse yourself in the world of fast and vivid vegetarian stir-fries. These dishes highlight a variety of colorful veggies, tofu, and lean protein, all beautifully seasoned and stir-fried to perfection. Experience the thrill of cooking nutritious and delectable meals in minutes, with the additional advantage of retaining the nutritional value of fresh ingredients.

Oven-Baked Goodness
Indulge in the warmth of oven-baked dishes that are both healthful and hearty. From roasted veggies to baked chicken and fish, these recipes employ the oven's magic to produce meals that are not only tasty but also simple to make. Uncover the secrets of generating golden crusts, luscious textures, and strong tastes.

Transform your nights with these healthful supper alternatives, delivering a great blend of nutrition and flavor. Whether you pick for lean protein dinners, vivid stir-fries, or oven-baked delights, these dishes promise to make your dinner table a place of sustenance and pleasure.

Guilt-Free Snacking

Explore the world of guilt-free eating with these healthful and enjoyable alternatives. From nutrient-packed nut and seed mixes to crispy vegetable chips with tasty dips, and delectable fruit-focused delights, this chapter offers snacks that support your body while pleasing your taste buds.

Nut and Seed Mixes
Elevate your snacking experience with a range of nut and seed mixes that give a perfect combination of good fats, protein, and critical elements.
Discover unique combinations, from spicy roasted almonds to antioxidant-rich trail mixes, ensuring your snack time is not only tasty but also nutritionally helpful.

Veggie Chips and Dips
Ditch the typical munchies for colorful and crispy vegetable chips combined with tasty dips. Explore oven-baked options to fulfill your appetite for a satisfying crunch,

and mix them with dips that vary from creamy hummus to yogurt-based treats. These combos provide a guilt-free and delightful way to munch throughout the day.

Fruit-Focused Treats
Indulge your sweet craving with fruit-focused delights that are not only tasty but also healthful. From frozen fruit popsicles to yogurt-covered berries, these dishes give a pleasant alternative to sugary snacking. Experience the natural sweetness of fruits while enjoying the extra advantages of vitamins and antioxidants.

Transform your snacking habits with these guilt-free choices. Whether you're grabbing for a nut and seed mix, diving into vegetable chips and dips, or relishing fruit-focused delights, these snacks are meant to keep you energetic and satiated between meals.

Beverages for Body Wellness

Quench your thirst and feed your body with a wonderful assortment of beverages meant to promote wellbeing. From hydrating infusions to nutrient-packed smoothies and herbal teas, this chapter discusses a range of beverages that will keep you refreshed and motivated throughout the day.

Hydrating Infusions
Stay hydrated with a twist by exploring our hydrating infusions. From citrus-infused water to herbal and floral combinations, these recipes make keeping hydrated a delightful experience. Discover unique combinations that not only refill your fluids but also give extra health advantages via natural components.

Nutrient-Packed Smoothies
Elevate your everyday nutrition with a range of nutrient-packed smoothies.

Explore vivid mixes of fruits, veggies, and superfoods that pander to your taste buds while offering a boost of vitamins and minerals. Whether you're searching for a morning pick-me-up or a post-workout refreshment, these smoothies have you covered.

Herbal Teas and Refreshing Drinks Unwind with a cup of herbal tea or enjoy a pleasant non-alcoholic beverage. Explore the world of herbal infusions and refreshing beverages that go beyond regular tea. From tranquil chamomile blends to stimulating mint mixtures, these recipes provide a soothing and health-conscious alternative to sugary drinks.

Revitalize your beverage selections with these alternatives created for bodily wellbeing. Whether you're sipping on hydrating infusions, mixing nutrient-packed smoothies, or savoring herbal teas, these drinks contribute to your entire well-being, making hydration a joyful and health-conscious experience.

Chapter three

Meal Planning and Prep

Efficiently manage your culinary journey with the skill of meal planning and preparation. This chapter includes practical recommendations for effective planning, discusses the ease of batch cooking, and offers inspired weekly menu ideas to simplify your approach to healthy and tasty meals.

Tips for Successful Planning
Master the art of meal planning with informative advice and tactics.

Learn how to construct balanced and diverse weekly meals, consider dietary preferences, and effectively arrange your grocery shopping. These strategies will enable you to keep on track with your dietary objectives while making meals a stress-free experience.

Batch Cooking for Convenience
Discover the simplicity of batch cooking as a time-saving technique for busy lives. Uncover the secrets of cooking bigger amounts of your favorite dishes, enabling you to have

healthful meals easily accessible throughout the week. Streamline your cooking procedure and enjoy the advantages of a well-stocked freezer and refrigerator.

Weekly Menu Ideas
Explore a selection of weekly food options that appeal to varied tastes and dietary demands. From themed dinner evenings to well-balanced meal plans, these ideas give inspiration for crafting different and pleasant weekly dinners. Find a rhythm that works for you and provides interest to your everyday meals.

Empower yourself with the skills to plan and cook meals effectively. Whether you're adopting helpful planning techniques, embracing batch cooking for convenience, or exploring new weekly meal ideas, this chapter offers you with the knowledge to make healthy eating a sustainable and pleasant part of your lifestyle.

Staying Motivated

Navigate the hurdles of maintaining a healthy lifestyle with techniques to remain motivated.

This chapter focuses on establishing realistic objectives, appreciating your accomplishments, and developing a sustainable basis for a healthy life.

Setting Realistic Goals
Define reasonable and meaningful health objectives targeted to your specific path. Learn how to create realistic targets that suit with your lifestyle, guaranteeing a feeling of success while minimizing unneeded pressure. Setting achievable objectives gives a blueprint for achievement and long-term commitment.

Celebrating Progress
Acknowledge and celebrate the milestones in your health path. Discover the value of celebrating successes, whether great or little, as they lead to continuous motivation. Celebrating success promotes healthy behaviors and encourages continuous devotion to your health and fitness objectives.

Building a Sustainable Healthy Lifestyle
Explore the aspects of a sustainable and balanced lifestyle. Learn how to incorporate healthy habits into your everyday routine,   making them a natural and permanent part of your life.

From mindful eating habits to regular physical exercise, maintaining a sustained healthy lifestyle guarantees that your well-being is a lifetime commitment.

Stay motivated on your road to health and wellbeing by using these tactics. Whether you're establishing realistic goals, celebrating victories, or developing a sustainable healthy lifestyle, this chapter offers as a guide to continuing your commitment to a happier and healthier self.

Chapter four

Section 2

Recipes ingredient and instruction

slim-down breakfast dishes together with their components and instructions:

1. Green Smoothie Bowl
Ingredients:
1 cup spinach
1/2 banana
1/2 cup pineapple chunks

1/2 cup almond milk
1 tbsp chia seeds
Toppings: sliced strawberries,
granola, and a sprinkle of honey.

Instructions:
1. Blend spinach, banana, pineapple,
and almond milk until smooth.
2. Pour into a bowl and top with sliced
strawberries, granola, and a drizzle of
honey.

2. Avocado Toast with Poached Egg
Ingredients:
1 piece whole-grain bread

1/2 avocado, mashed
1 poached egg
Salt and pepper to taste
Optional toppings: red pepper flakes,
cherry tomatoes.

Instructions:
1. Toast the bread slice.
2. Spread mashed avocado on the
bread.
3. Place the poached egg on top and
season with salt, pepper, and optional
garnishes.

3. Greek Yogurt Parfait
Ingredients:

1 cup Greek yogurt
1/2 cup mixed berries (blueberries,
raspberries, strawberries)
2 tablespoons granola
1 tablespoon honey

Instructions:
1. In a glass or dish, layer Greek
yogurt, mixed berries, and granola.
2. Drizzle honey over the top.

4. Quinoa Breakfast Bowl
Ingredients:
1/2 cup cooked quinoa
1/4 cup almond milk
1/2 apple, diced
1 tablespoon chopped nuts (e. g. ,

almonds or walnuts)
1 teaspoon honey

Instructions:
1. Mix cooked quinoa with almond milk.
2. Top with sliced apple, chopped nuts, and a drizzle of honey.
5. Chia Seed Pudding
Ingredients:
2 teaspoons chia seeds
1/2 cup almond milk
1/4 teaspoon vanilla extract
Fresh berries for topping

Instructions:
1. Mix chia seeds, almond milk, and vanilla essence in a container.
2. Refrigerate overnight.
3. Top with fresh berries before serving.

6. Oatmeal with Nut Butter
Ingredients:
1/2 cup oats
1 cup water or milk
1 tablespoon almond butter or peanut butter
Sliced banana for topping

Instructions:
1. Cook oats with water or milk.

2. Stir in nut butter until fully blended.

3. Top with sliced banana.

7. Egg White Veggie Omelette

Ingredients:

3 egg whites

1/4 cup chopped bell peppers

1/4 cup chopped tomatoes

Handful of spinach

Salt and pepper to taste

Instructions:

1. Whisk egg whites and pour into a hot, non-stick pan.

2. Add vegetables, season with salt and pepper, and fold into an omelette.

8. Whole Grain Pancakes
Ingredients:
1/2 cup whole grain flour
1/2 cup almond milk
1 teaspoon baking powder
1 tablespoon honey
Fresh berries for topping

Instructions:
1. Mix flour, almond milk, baking powder, and honey.
2. Cook pancakes on a griddle.
3. Top with fresh berries.

9. Turkey and Veggie Breakfast Wrap
Ingredients:
1 whole-grain wrap

2 slices turkey
1 scrambled egg
Salsa or spicy sauce for taste
Handful of spinach

Instructions:
1. Layer turkey slices, scrambled egg, and spinach on the wrap.
2. Add salsa or spicy sauce for added flavor.
3. Roll up and enjoy.

10. Coconut and Berry Smoothie
Ingredients:
1/2 cup coconut water
1/2 cup coconut milk

1/2 cup mixed berries (strawberries, blueberries, raspberries)
1 tablespoon shredded coconut

Instructions:
1. Blend coconut water, coconut milk, and mixed berries until smooth.
2. Pour into a glass and add shredded coconut on top.

slim-down lunch meals together with their components and instructions:

1. Quinoa Salad with Grilled Chicken
Ingredients:

1 cup cooked quinoa
Grilled chicken breast strips
Cherry tomatoes, halved
Cucumber, diced
Feta cheese crumbles
Balsamic vinaigrette dressing

Instructions:
1. In a bowl, mix quinoa, grilled chicken, cherry tomatoes, cucumber, and feta.
2. Drizzle with balsamic vinaigrette and stir gently.

2. Mediterranean Chickpea Bowl
Ingredients:

1 cup cooked chickpeas
Cherry tomatoes, sliced
Cucumber, diced
Kalamata olives, sliced
Red onion, finely chopped
Feta cheese crumbles
Olive oil and lemon dressing

Instructions:
1. Combine chickpeas, tomatoes, cucumber, olives, red onion, and feta in a bowl.
2. Drizzle with olive oil and lemon dressing.

3. Salmon and Quinoa Stuffed Bell Peppers

Ingredients:
Bell peppers, half
Cooked quinoa
Baked or grilled salmon, flakes
Spinach, chopped
Lemon zest
Dill, chopped

Instructions:
1. Stuff bell peppers with a blend of
quinoa, salmon, spinach, lemon
zest, and dill.
2. Bake until peppers are soft.

4. Veggie Wrap with Hummus
Ingredients:

Whole-grain wrap
Hummus
Mixed vegetables (bell peppers,
cucumber, carrot, spinach)
Avocado slices
Feta cheese (optional)

Instructions:
1. Spread hummus on the wrap.
2. Add mixed vegetables, avocado
slices, and optional feta.
3. Roll up and slice.

5. Shrimp and Quinoa Stir-Fry
Ingredients:
Shrimp, peeled and deveined
Quinoa, cooked

Broccoli florets
Bell peppers, sliced
Soy sauce
Ginger with garlic, minced

Instructions:
1. Stir-fry shrimp, broccoli, and bell
peppers in a skillet with ginger and
garlic.
2. Mix in cooked quinoa and soy sauce.

6. Caprese Salad with Grilled Chicken
Ingredients:
Grilled chicken breast
Tomato slices
Fresh mozzarella, sliced

Fresh basil leaves
Balsamic glaze
Olive oil

Instructions:
1. Arrange grilled chicken, tomato, mozzarella, and basil on a platter.
2. Drizzle with balsamic glaze and olive oil.

7. Black Bean and Corn Salad
#Ingredients:
Black beans, canned and drained
Corn kernels, cooked
Red onion, finely chopped
Cilantro, chopped

Lime juice
Salt and pepper to taste

Instructions:
1. Mix black beans, corn, red onion,
and cilantro in a bowl.
2. Squeeze lime juice over the salad
and season with salt and pepper.

8. Turkey and Veggie Lettuce Wraps
Ingredients:
Lean ground turkey
Lettuce leaves
Tomatoes, diced
Avocado, sliced
Greek yogurt (as a topping)
Cumin and chili powder (for flavoring)

Instructions:
1. Cook ground turkey with cumin and chili powder.
2. Spoon turkey onto lettuce leaves and top with tomatoes, avocado, and a dollop of Greek yogurt.

9. Sweet Potato and Chickpea Buddha Bowl
Ingredients:
Roasted sweet potato cubes
Cooked chickpeas
Quinoa, cooked
Kale, rubbed with olive oil
Tahini dressing

Instructions:
 1. Arrange sweet potato, chickpeas, quinoa, and spinach in a bowl.
2. Drizzle with tahini dressing.

10. Cauliflower Fried Rice with Tofu
Ingredients:
Cauliflower rice
Extra-firm tofu, cubed
Mixed veggies (peas, carrots, corn)
Soy sauce
Sesame oil
Scallions, chopped

Instructions:
1. Sauté tofu and mixed veggies in sesame oil.

2. Add cauliflower rice and soy sauce, simmer until heated through.
3. Garnish with sliced scallions.

These lunch ideas provide a range of tastes and nutrients to keep you satiated and energetic throughout the day. Adjust quantities according on your nutritional requirements and tastes.

Chapter five

1. Baked Lemon Herb Salmon
Ingredients:
Salmon fillets
Lemon juice
Fresh herbs (rosemary, thyme)
Garlic, minced
Olive oil
Salt and pepper

Instructions:
1. Preheat the oven. Place salmon fillets on a baking sheet.
2. Drizzle with lemon juice, olive oil, sprinkle herbs and chopped garlic.
3. Bake until the fish is cooked through.

2. Vegetarian Zucchini Noodles with Pesto
Ingredients:
Zucchini noodles
Cherry tomatoes, halved
Basil pesto
Pine nuts
Parmesan cheese (optional)

Instructions:
1. Spiralize zucchini into noodles.
2. Toss with cherry tomatoes, pesto, and pine nuts.
3. Garnish with Parmesan if desired.

3. Grilled Chicken and Veggie Skewers
Ingredients:
Chicken breast, diced
Bell peppers, onions, cherry tomatoes
Olive oil
Lemon juice
Italian seasoning
Salt and pepper

Instructions:
1. Thread chicken and vegetables onto skewers.
2. Mix olive oil, lemon juice, Italian seasoning, salt, and pepper.
3. Grill skewers until chicken is done.

4. Stuffed Bell Peppers with Turkey and Quinoa
Ingredients:
Bell peppers, half
Ground turkey
Quinoa, cooked
Black beans, drained
Salsa
Mexican mix cheese

Instructions:
1. Brown turkey, combine with quinoa, black beans, and salsa.
2. Stuff bell peppers, cover with cheese, then bake until cheese is melted.

5. Shrimp and Asparagus Stir-Fry
Ingredients:
Shrimp, peeled and deveined
Asparagus, chopped
Garlic, minced
Soy sauce
Sesame oil
Red pepper flakes

Instructions:
1. Stir-fry shrimp and asparagus with garlic in sesame oil.
2. Add soy sauce and red pepper flakes.

6. Eggplant Parmesan
Ingredients:
Eggplant, sliced
Marinara sauce
Mozzarella cheese
Parmesan cheese
Bread crumbs
Olive oil

Instructions:
1. Dip eggplant slices in breadcrumbs and bake until brown.

2. Layer with marinara sauce and cheeses. Bake until bubbling.

7. Cauliflower and Broccoli Alfredo Pasta
Ingredients:
Cauliflower florets
Broccoli florets
Whole-grain pasta
Almond milk
Parmesan cheese
Garlic powder

Instructions:
1. Boil cauliflower and broccoli till soft.
2. Blend with almond milk, Parmesan, and garlic powder.
3. Toss with cooked spaghetti.

8. Teriyaki Tofu Stir-Fry
Ingredients:
Extra-firm tofu, cubed
Mixed veggies (broccoli, bell peppers,
snap peas)
Teriyaki sauce
Brown rice

Instructions:
1. Sauté tofu and vegetables, add
teriyaki sauce.
2. Serve over cooked brown rice.

9. Turkey and Vegetable Lettuce Wraps
Ingredients:
Lean ground turkey

Lettuce leaves
Stir-fried veggies (bell peppers,
carrots, water chestnuts)
Hoisin sauce

Instructions:
1. Cook turkey, add stir-fried
vegetables and hoisin sauce.
2. Spoon into lettuce leaves.

10. Chickpea and Spinach Curry
Ingredients:
Chickpeas, canned and drained
Spinach
Coconut milk
Curry powder

Garlic, minced
Brown rice

Instructions:
1. Sauté garlic, add chickpeas, spinach, coconut milk, and curry spice.
2. Simmer till heated through. Serve over brown rice.

These supper dishes offer a variety of tastes and nutrients to help you relax and replenish at the end of the day. Adjust quantities according on your nutritional requirements and tastes.

healthful and slim-down snack recipes together with their components and instructions:

1. Greek Yogurt and Berry Parfait
Ingredients:
Greek yogurt
Mixed berries (blueberries, strawberries, raspberries)
Granola
Honney

Instructions:
1. In a glass or dish, layer Greek yogurt with mixed berries and granola.

2. Drizzle with honey for sweetness.

2. Roasted Chickpeas
Ingredients:
Canned chickpeas, rinsed and dried
Olive oil
Smoked paprika
Garlic powder
Salt

Instructions:
1. Toss chickpeas with olive oil, smoked paprika, garlic powder, and salt.
2. Roast in the oven until crispy.

3. Apple Slices with Almond Butter
Ingredients: Apple, sliced Almond
butter

 Instructions: 1. Spread almond butter
over apple slices for a delightful crunch.

4. Veggie Sticks with Hummus
 Ingredients: Carrot, cucumber, and
bell pepper sticks
 Hummus

Instructions: 1. Dip carrot sticks into
hummus for a healthful and crispy
snack.

5.   Dark Chocolate and Almond Trail Mix

Ingredients:
Dark chocolate chunks
Almonds
Dried cranberries
Pumpkin seeds

Instructions:
1. Mix dark chocolate pieces with almonds, dried cranberries, and pumpkin seeds.

6.   Cottage Cheese and Pineapple Bowl

Ingredients:
Cottage cheese
Fresh pineapple chunks
Mint leaves (optional)

Instructions:

1. Combine cottage cheese with fresh pineapple pieces.
2. Garnish with mint leaves for a refreshing twist.

7. Kale Chips Ingredients: Fresh kale, stems removed

Olive oil

Nutritional yeast Sea salt

Instructions:

1. Toss kale with olive oil, nutritional yeast, and sea salt.
2. Bake until crispy for a guilt-free chip substitute.

8. Banana and Peanut Butter Bites

Ingredients: Banana, sliced Peanut butter

Instructions: 1. Spread peanut butter over banana slices for a fast and tasty snack.

9. Chia Seed Pudding with Berries

Ingredients: Chia seeds
 Almond milk Mixed berries (strawberries, blueberries, raspberries)

Instructions:
1. Mix chia seeds with almond milk and chill until thick.

2. Top with mixed berries before serving.

10. Rice Cake with Avocado and Cherry Tomatoes
Ingredients: Brown rice cake Avocado, mashed Cherry tomatoes, sliced Salt & pepper

Instructions:
1. Spread mashed avocado on a rice cake.
2. Top with sliced cherry tomatoes, salt, and pepper.

These snack dishes provide a blend of nutrients and tastes to keep you pleased between meals.

excellent seafood and fish dishes together with their components and instructions:

1. **Lemon Garlic Butter Shrimp**
Ingredient Shrimp, peeled and deveined Butter Garlic, minced Lemon juice
Fresh parsley, chopped

 Instructions:
1. In a pan, melt butter over medium heat.
2. Add minced garlic and sauté till fragrant.

3. Add shrimp, heat until they become pink.

4. Squeeze lemon juice over shrimp and sprinkle with fresh parsley.

5. Toss to coat and serve over rice or spaghetti.

2. Grilled Salmon with Dill Sauce
Ingredients:
Salmon fillets
Olive oil Lemon juice
Dill, chopped Greek yogurt
Salt and pepper

Instructions:
1. Brush fish with olive oil and season with salt and pepper.

2. Grill until cooked thoroughly.

3. Mix chopped dill, Greek yogurt,
and lemon juice for the sauce.
4. Serve grilled fish with the dill sauce.

3. Tuna and Avocado Salad

Ingredients: Canned tuna, drained
Avocado, diced Red onion, finely
chopped Cherry tomatoes, halved
Cilantro, chopped Lime juice
Salt and pepper

Instructions:
1. Mix tuna, avocado, red onion,
cherry tomatoes, and cilantro in a
bowl.
2. Drizzle with lime juice and season
with salt and pepper.

3. Toss gently and serve over
whole-grain crackers or as a salad.

4. Garlic Herb Baked Cod
Ingredients:
Cod fillets
Olive oil
Garlic, minced
Fresh herbs (rosemary, thyme)
Lemon slices
Salt and pepper

Instructions:
1. Preheat the oven. Place fish fillets
on a baking sheet.

2. Drizzle with olive oil, add minced garlic, fresh herbs, and season with salt and pepper.

3. Top with lemon slices.

4. Bake until the fish is flaky and cooked thoroughly.

5. **Mango Salsa Shrimp Tacos**

Ingredients: Shrimp, peeled and deveined Corn or whole-grain tortillas Mango, diced Red onion, finely chopped Cilantro, chopped Lime juice Chili powder

Greek yogurt (optional for topping)

Instructions:
1. Sauté shrimp with chili powder until cooked.

2. In a bowl, combine chopped mango, red onion, cilantro, and lime juice to create salsa.
3. Warm tortillas and fill with shrimp and mango salsa.
4. Optionally, top with a dollop of Greek yogurt.

These seafood and fish dishes provide a range of tastes and are high in omega-3 fatty acids and lean protein. Adjust quantities according on your nutritional requirements and tastes.

Chapter six

Delicious meat dishes together with their ingredients and instructions:

1. Balsamic Glazed Chicken Breast
Ingredients:
 Chicken breasts
 Balsamic vinegar
Olive oil
Garlic, minced
 Dried thyme
 Salt and pepper

Instructions:
1. Season chicken breasts with salt, pepper, and dried thyme.
2. In a pan, saute chicken breasts until brown.
3. Mix balsamic vinegar, olive oil, and minced garlic.
4. Pour the balsamic mixture over the chicken and boil until the glaze thickens.

2. Beef and Vegetable Stir-Fry
Ingredients:
Beef sirloin strips
Mixed veggies (broccoli, bell peppers, snap peas)

Soy sauce
Sesame oil
Ginger, minced
Garlic, minced
Brown rice

Instructions:
1. Stir-fry meat until browned.
Remove from the pan.
2. Stir-fry veggies with ginger and
garlic.
3. Add back the steak, add soy sauce
and sesame oil.
4. Serve over cooked brown rice.

3. Herb-Crusted Pork Tenderloin

Ingredients:

Pork tenderloin
Dijon mustard
Fresh herbs (rosemary, thyme)
Garlic, minced Olive oil
Salt and pepper

Instructions:
1. Preheat the oven. Rub pork with
Dijon mustard, chopped garlic, and
fresh herbs.
2. Sear in a pan with olive oil.
3. Roast in the oven until meat
achieves the desired doneness.

4. Turkey and Quinoa Stuffed Peppers
Ingredients: Ground turkey Quinoa,
cooked Bell peppers, halved Onion,
diced Tomato sauce
 Italian seasoning
 Mozzarella cheese

 Instructions:
1. Cook turkey with chopped onion
until browned.
2. Mix with cooked quinoa, Italian
seasoning, and tomato sauce.
3. Stuff bell peppers, cover with
mozzarella, and bake until cheese
melts.

5. Lemon Herb Grilled Lamb Chops

Ingredients: Lamb chops
 Lemon zest Fresh mint, chopped
Garlic, minced Olive oil
Salt and pepper

 Instructions:
1. Combine lemon zest, chopped mint,
minced garlic, olive oil, salt, and
pepper.
2. Coat lamb chops with the mixture.
3. Grill until lamb gets the desired
doneness.

These meat dishes provide a diversity
of tastes and cooking methods to keep
your dinners fascinating.

Adjust quantities according on your nutritional requirements and tastes.

pleasant fruit-based drinks together with their ingredients and instructions:

1. Watermelon Mint Cooler
Ingredients: Watermelon, diced
Fresh mint leaves
Lime juice
Sparkling water

Instructions:
1. Blend watermelon cubes till smooth.
2. Strain the juice to eliminate pulp.
3. Mix with fresh mint leaves,

lime juice, and sparkling water.
4. Serve over ice.

2. Berry Citrus Smoothie
Ingredients:
Mixed berries (strawberries,
blueberries, raspberries) Orange juice
 Greek yogurt
Honey

Instructions:
1. Blend mixed berries with orange
juice and Greek yogurt.
2. Sweeten with honey to taste.
3. Blend until smooth and serve.

 3. Pineapple Coconut Refresher
Ingredients:

Pineapple chunks
Coconut water
Lime juice
Ice cubes

Instructions:
1. Blend pineapple chunks with coconut water and lime juice.
2. Strain the mixture.
3. Serve over ice for a tropical refreshment.

4. Cucumber Mint Infused Water
Ingredients: Cucumber, sliced Fresh mint leaves Water

Instructions: 1. Combine cucumber slices and fresh mint leaves in a pitcher.
2. Fill the pitcher with water and chill for a few hours.
3. Serve over ice for a hydrating and refreshing beverage.

5. Mango Basil Iced Tea
Ingredients: Black tea bags
Hot water
Mango, diced
Fresh basil leaves
Honey (optional)
Instructions:
1. Brew black tea with hot water and let it cool.

2. Blend diced mango until smooth.
3. Mix mango puree with the cooled tea.
4. Add fresh basil leaves and sweeten with honey if desired.
5. Serve over ice for a delicious iced tea.

These fruit-based drinks deliver a burst of tastes and are excellent for keeping hydrated. Adjust sweetness and ingredients according on your taste preferences.

colorful salad dishes with a range of tastes and textures

1. Caprese Salad with Balsamic Glaze
Ingredients: Fresh tomatoes, sliced
Fresh mozzarella, sliced
Fresh basil leaves
Balsamic glaze
Olive oil
Salt and pepper

Instructions:
1. Arrange tomato and mozzarella slices on a platter.
2. Tuck fresh basil leaves between the slices.
3. Drizzle with balsamic glaze and olive oil.

4. Sprinkle with salt and pepper to taste.

2. Mango Avocado Quinoa Salad

Ingredients: Cooked quinoa
 Ripe mango, diced Avocado, diced
Red onion, finely chopped Cilantro,
chopped Lime juice
 Salt and pepper

nstructions: 1. In a bowl, mix quinoa,
mango, avocado, red onion, and
cilantro.
2. Squeeze lime juice over the salad.
3. Season with salt and pepper to taste.

3. Greek Salad with Tzatziki Dressing

Ingredients: Cucumbers, diced Cherry tomatoes, halved Kalamata olives, sliced Feta cheese, crumbled Red onion, thinly sliced Tzatziki dressing

Instructions:
1. Mix cucumbers, cherry tomatoes, olives, feta, and red onion in a bowl.
2. Drizzle with tzatziki dressing and stir gently.

4. Kale and Quinoa Salad with Lemon Vinaigrette
Ingredients: Kale, chopped
 Cooked quinoa
Cherry tomatoes, halved Pomegranate seeds

Feta cheese, crumbled
Lemon vinaigrette

Instructions:
1. Massage greens with lemon
vinaigrette until soft.
2. Toss with quinoa, cherry tomatoes,
pomegranate seeds, and feta.

5. Chicken and Berry Salad with Poppy
Seed Dressing
Ingredients:
Grilled chicken breast, sliced
Mixed greens
Strawberries, sliced Blueberries
Goat cheese, crumbled
Candied pecans
Poppy seed dressing

Instructions:
1. Arrange mixed greens on a platter.
2. Top with grilled chicken, strawberries, blueberries, goat cheese, and candied pecans.
3. Drizzle with poppy seed dressing.

These salad dishes give a blend of textures and tastes, making them both pleasant and healthful. Adjust ingredients and amounts according on your tastes.

excellent vegetable dishes that demonstrate a range of cooking methods and flavors:

1. Roasted Vegetable Medley
Ingredients:
 Assorted veggies (bell peppers,
zucchini, cherry tomatoes, carrots)
Olive oil
Garlic, minced Italian seasoning
Salt and pepper

 Instructions:
1. Preheat the oven. Toss chopped
veggies with olive oil, minced garlic,
Italian seasoning, salt, and pepper.
2. Roast in the oven until veggies are
soft and slightly browned.

2. Stir-Fried Broccoli and Snow Peas
Ingredients:
Broccoli florets

Snow peas, trimmed Garlic, minced
Soy sauce
Sesame oil
Red pepper flakes

 Instructions:
1. In a wok or skillet, stir-fry broccoli
and snow peas with chopped garlic in
sesame oil.
2. Add soy sauce and red pepper flakes
for taste.

3. Zucchini Noodles with Pesto
 Ingredients: Zucchini, spiralized into
noodles
Cherry tomatoes, halved Pesto sauce
 Pine nuts Parmesan cheese (optional)

Instructions:
1. Sauté zucchini noodles and cherry tomatoes until just soft.
2. Toss with pesto sauce.
3. Top with pine nuts and Parmesan if preferred.

4. Cauliflower and Chickpea Curry
Ingredients:
Cauliflower florets
 Chickpeas, canned and drained Onion, chopped Tomato, diced Curry powder
 Coconut milk
 Cilantro, chopped

Instructions:

1. Sauté chopped onion till transparent.

2. Add cauliflower, chickpeas, chopped tomato, curry powder, and coconut milk.

3. Simmer until cauliflower is soft. Garnish with cilantro.

5. Baked Stuffed Bell Peppers
Ingredients: Bell peppers, halved
Quinoa, cooked Black beans, canned and drained Corn kernels
 Salsa Mexican mix cheese
Avocado, diced (for topping)

Instructions:
1. Mix cooked quinoa, black beans, corn, and salsa.
2. Stuff bell peppers with the mixture, top with cheese.
3. Bake until peppers are soft.
4. Garnish with chopped avocado before serving.

These vegetable dishes provide a range of tastes and health advantages. Adjust ingredients and spices according to your taste preferences.

wonderful dessert recipes to fulfill your sweet tooth:

1. Berry Parfait with Greek Yogurt
Ingredients:
Greek yogurt
Mixed berries (strawberries, blueberries, raspberries)
Honey Granola

Instructions:
1. In a glass, layer Greek yogurt, mixed berries, and granola.
2. Drizzle honey over the top for sweetness.

2.   Chocolate Avocado Mousse
Ingredients: Ripe avocados
Cocoa powder
 Maple syrup or honey
Vanilla extract Almond milk

 Instructions:
1. Blend avocados, cocoa powder,
maple syrup, vanilla extract, and
almond milk until smooth.
2. Chill in the refrigerator before
serving.

3. Baked Apple with Cinnamon and
Almonds
Ingredients: Apples, cored and halved
Cinnamon Almonds, chopped Honey

Instructions:
1. Place apple halves on a baking sheet.
2. Sprinkle with cinnamon and
chopped almonds.
3. Drizzle honey over the top.
4. Bake until apples are soft.

 4. Chia Seed Pudding with Mango
 Ingredients:
Chia seeds
Almond milk
 Mango, diced Coconut flakes

Instructions:
1. Mix chia seeds with almond milk and
chill until thick.
2. Layer with chopped mango and top
with coconut flakes.

5. Banana and Walnut Baked Oatmeal
Ingredients:
 Rolled oats Ripe bananas, mashed
Walnuts, chopped Maple syrup
 Almond milk
Vanilla extract
 Instructions:
1. Mix rolled oats, mashed bananas,
chopped walnuts, maple syrup,
almond milk, and vanilla extract.
2. Bake until the top is brown and
crispy.

These dessert dishes provide a blend of
tastes and textures while combining
nutritional ingredients. Adjust
sweetness and ingredients according to
your tastes. The

www.ingramcontent.com/pod-product-compliance
Lightning Source LLC
Chambersburg PA
CBHW070743250726
48662CB00004B/1624